Moving Moments

Romances for Seniors

seniorality

Moving Moments -
Jamie Stonebridge, Stacy J Roberts

Copyright © 2024
Seniorality / Everbreeze Media Oy

This is a work of fiction. Names and characters are the product of the author's imagination and any resemblance to actual persons, living or dead, is entirely coincidental.

Set in 22 pt EB Garamond

Chapter 1
A New Beginning

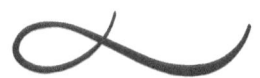

SARAH pulled into the driveway, sitting in the car for a moment as she took in her new home. It was a blisteringly hot summer's day and the top of her convertible was down. The young woman gazed at the house with a broad grin.

She somehow knew that the move to Florida marked the beginning of a positive new chapter in her life. She just hoped she could adjust to the unaccustomed humidity.

Sarah had squealed with joy when she was offered a teaching job in Weston. Not only did it mean living closer to her retired parents, but who could resist the inviting Florida sunshine?

Even so, the twenty-six-year-old was still nervous about this new challenge. Teaching a class here would be such a contrast to teaching in the remote town of her native Michigan.

Back home, the classes were small, and all the families knew one another. Here, it was sure to be different. There would definitely be more children, but could she establish the same closeness with her pupils that she had in her old school? Only time would tell.

"I can't believe I managed to get this place; it's perfect," she said to herself while slipping out from behind the wheel, excited to explore her new home.

The house featured a meticulously manicured lawn bordered by beds filled with a variety of colorful flowers. Tall palms loomed overhead, offering only a hint of shade from the midday sun as she walked beneath them.

She followed the path to the front door, pausing to take a deep breath before unlocking it for the first time.

When Sarah had met the realtor a month ago to view the property, she was stunned to discover that she could easily afford the place. However, she knew it had more to do with her father's friendship with the agency owner handling the lease, rather than anything else.

Yet, for once, she was content to take advantage of his generosity to be able to live in such a lovely neighborhood.

She strolled around the house, whisking away the dust sheets that covered the furniture. Bright sunlight streamed into every room as she drew back the drapes, immediately opening the windows to allow a light breeze to drift through the property.

The open-plan kitchen boasted mahogany units, but the floor-to-ceiling windows in the adjoining dining area brightened the dark colors. It certainly had style. Pulling open the patio doors, Sarah stepped onto the deck.

She sighed heavily, catching the welcome sight of the plunge pool, its cool water sparkling temptingly in the sunshine.

Even though she had opted for denim shorts and a light flowery top, Sarah was beginning to feel the effects of the

Florida heat, as tiny beads of perspiration were forming on her brow.

"Later, definitely," she promised herself.

Heading back out front, she opened the trunk of her car. Before Sarah could collect any of the boxes, a voice called out, "Hi there. Are you moving in?"

Sarah turned to see a slim brunette striding toward her. She wore a short floral dress with spaghetti straps, and not an inch of white flesh showed upon her tanned skin. The stranger held out a slender hand with immaculately manicured nails.

"I'm Zoe," she said as she introduced herself.

"I'm Sarah, and yes, I am moving in."

"Sorry for being so nosy, but not much goes on around here," Zoe chuckled.

"It looks like a lovely neighborhood," Sarah observed as she glanced up and down the street.

The sound of children's laughter drifted toward the women from a nearby backyard. Aromas from a barbecue wafted through the air, making both their stomachs rumble hungrily.

"To be honest, I couldn't imagine living anywhere else. Tom and I moved in ten years ago and haven't been happier," said Zoe.

With a warm smile, Zoe lightly touched Sarah's arm as she insisted, "Listen, leave all that for now. It's too hot to be lugging those boxes about. Come across the road and I will get you a glass of iced tea."

Relieved by the offer, Sarah admitted that she could use something to quench her thirst. However, she still eyed her belongings with a sense of guilt as she re-locked the trunk.

"Don't you worry about unpacking," Zoe stated matter-of-factually.

Sarah's frown turned into a smile as her new friend explained, "I have two teenage sons, so they can carry your things in from the car, when they get home from school."

And with that, she gave a cheeky wink before beginning to giggle. As Zoe linked arms at that moment with Sarah, Sarah knew they would become close friends. The woman was like a breath of fresh air, chattering happily as she steered them toward her house.

"Wow!" Sarah gasped.

Zoe smiled proudly, saying, "Welcome to my oasis."

The backyard was occupied mainly by a full-sized swimming pool with diving boards at the far end. However, the rest of the ground was covered with a lush green lawn. Several loungers were scattered around, and a row of thick firs and palms secluded the whole area.

Flopping down on one of the seats, Zoe began to pour some iced tea. Cubes of ice clinked against the tall glass, and Sarah smiled as she accepted the drink.

"So, what brings you to Weston?" Zoe asked politely, as the two women settled in the shade, out of the blazing sun.

"I start work at the local elementary school in the new semester," Sarah explained.

"Oh, that's great. Some of your pupils actually live on this street."

As Zoe began to list the numerous local families, Sarah absorbed every detail, aware that the more she knew, the easier it would be when she finally got to meet them all.

The whole street appeared to be like its own little community, where everyone seemed to be friends. This was just the sort of place Sarah had always wanted to live.

"Do you work at all?" Sarah asked curiously.

A brief frown creased her brow as Zoe began to chuckle, until the other woman told her, "My dear, I played it smart. I married a man who works in finance in the city. I have grown quite accustomed to my life of leisure, now that the boys are older."

With that, the woman began to tell her all about her shopping trips, lunches with friends in a local gin bar and luxury days at the local spa. Although Sarah felt envious at first, she was quick to realize that she would soon become bored with such a lifestyle over time.

"I used to work as a legal secretary and offered to return to work once the boys started school. But, Tom wanted me to be here when they got home."

"That must be nice for you," Sarah answered politely.

"Ah, and here they are!" Zoe suddenly declared.

Turning her head, Sarah saw two teenage boys coming round the corner of the house. Both of them looked uncomfortable in the uniform they had to wear - the stiff shirt and shorts were clearly not designed for the warm weather.

After kissing their mother's cheek, they flopped beside her on the lounger. Each one gulped down the cold drink Zoe poured for them before she introduced her guest.

Sarah smiled as the boys excused themselves after politely shaking her hand. She watched as they disappeared into the house to freshen up and change into something cooler.

"You must be very proud of them."

"I am," Zoe beamed - her love for her sons was evident.

The boys didn't utter a word of complaint when, a little later, their mother asked them to move Sarah's belongings from her car. Their help meant that she had all her things inside the house in no time at all.

Setting down the box she had carried, Zoe flexed her arms before saying, "Well, I think that's the last one."

"Thank you so much," Sarah said gratefully.

"Oh, it's no bother at all". Said Zoe, "Now, are you sure you won't join us for dinner later when Tom gets home?"

"No, really, but thank you for the offer. I just have so much to sort out here."

Sarah swept her arm around the lounge, which was now cluttered with bags and boxes.

"I understand. But you're welcome over the road if you change your mind."

However, once Zoe and her sons left, Sarah went straight to work. She dug out her portable radio and tuned it to her favorite station, humming along to the tunes as she began to unpack and organize her belongings.

The young woman barely noticed the sundown as she gave everything its place, only realizing how late it had gotten when she finally sat down on the couch with an exhausted sigh.

Sarah realized she couldn't properly relax yet. She headed to her en-suite bathroom, hopped into the shower, and happily lathered the sweetly fragranced suds over her body, scrubbing away the day's sweat until she was completely refreshed.

Sarah settled in the lounge after slipping into a pair of pink satin pajamas. Music was still playing softly in the background as she sipped the wine she had treated herself with.

A loud rap at the door startled her slightly, and quickly, she pulled on a robe before opening the door just a crack.

Zoe stood on the stoop, her arms laden with plates of food. "Listen, I remember what it was like when we moved in. The last thing you want to do on your first night is to start preparing food. So, I thought I would put some dinner on one side for you. It's just a simple chicken salad, nothing fancy."

"That is so kind of you," Sarah gushed with real appreciation.

At last, all the stress and tension she had felt due to the move left her. Feeling more settled than she had in years, Sarah knew that the change from Michigan to Florida had led her to a place she could call home.

Chapter 2
A Fortunate Encounter

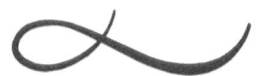

AFTER reluctantly climbing out from beneath the soft cotton sheets, Sarah opened the bedroom drapes. The morning sunlight immediately brightened the room, even though it was still early.

As a teacher, she was used to waking at this hour. She still yawned as she headed down to the kitchen, flicking on the coffee maker before pulling up the blind.

The window looked out over the backyard, but the low bordering hedge allowed her to see into her neighbor's property.

A small dark-haired boy was still wearing his dinosaur pajamas and quietly playing in the sandpit.

"That must be Curtis," Sarah muttered aloud.

Zoe had told Sarah all she knew about the Jackson family yesterday, informing her that the father, Mike, had bought the house just last year. He remained somewhat of a mystery, although Zoe had heard that he was a mechanic.

"Now I'm a married woman, of course," Zoe had said. "But, if I wasn't... well..."

Sarah had laughed along with her friend, but the comment had left her curious about her new neighbor.

Suddenly, there he was. A tall man with short-cropped brown hair and a bare torso that clearly showed he spent time at the gym. She couldn't see his face, but admired his rippling muscles as the stranger picked up his son and carried him inside.

"Well, Zoe was right. He's certainly not bad 'eye candy'," she chuckled.

But men were the last thing on the young woman's mind. She had left a relationship behind in Michigan that had become so stifling. She was certainly in no rush to get back onto the dating scene anytime soon.

Sarah sat outside on the rear deck with a mug of fresh coffee in her hand. She opened a copy of the local paper that she had retrieved from her front step earlier.

"Wow!" she gasped while scanning through the pages.

Each one had advertisements for various upcoming events and the majority of them, family-oriented. It was such a lovely sight to see all the competitions and activities that were organized for the children during the school holidays.

Yet, it seemed like no one had been left out. There were numerous activities for everyone in the community to enjoy. Sarah was keen to offer her help and get involved once she was settled.

When her parents retired to Weston five years ago, Sarah had been eager to follow. However, she had commitments to the school that employed her and had to wait for her contract to end.

When she spotted the ad for a teacher in Florida, it was like all her prayers had been answered. Mom and Dad had always told her about the neighborly feel of the place, and even though she had only been there one day, Sarah already had a sense that they were right.

After another boost of caffeine, she jumped into the shower before pulling on a fresh pair of shorts and a strappy red T-shirt. She cursed loudly when she stubbed her bare toe against one of the remaining boxes in the hall.

Yesterday had been a long day, and once she finished unpacking in the house, she couldn't muster the energy to move some things to the garage. Each box was clearly marked as "tools" or "decorating"- her dad's idea, so she was always prepared. But, they didn't need to be in the house.

She laced her sneakers before lifting the first box, grunting at the weight. The garage door slid open with a simple touch of her elbow, and she nodded, impressed.

Luckily, the property owners had installed rows of wooden shelving along the back wall of the garage. Sarah began to fill them with things that could just be stored until they were needed.

"Wow! I don't think I will need the gym later," she mumbled to herself.

Sarah could feel the strain in her arms as she lifted the last box. With a groan, she raised it higher, trying to slide it into an empty space. Finally, she had finished and was looking forward to a cool drink.

"What the?" she suddenly squealed.

A man had appeared from nowhere, reaching above her head and deftly catching the box she had just placed from falling and hitting her on the head. She looked up at him gratefully, recognizing the stranger as her neighbor next door.

"Thank you."

"It's all right," he answered with a grin that showed a small dimple on his right cheek.

He took her hand and gave it a firm shake as he said, "I'm Mike Jackson, from number 230."

"Sarah Willis. And thanks again for saving me from that rogue box. I didn't even see you come in."

"I've just dropped my son off at his friend's house for a play-date, so it was lucky I was passing," he said.

Their eyes were locked and Sarah struggled to avert her stare. Mike's eyes were the brightest shade of emerald green she had ever seen. She knew that if she didn't look away, she would drown in their depths. They sparkled now as she stammered her words.

"Would, you, erm, like a drink? I have soda in the cooler. Just my way of repaying your kindness."

Mike accepted her offer and she felt surprisingly restless as she led him through to the kitchen. With her back to him, Sarah opened the cooler door, relieved as the chilled air hit her skin and grateful that he couldn't see her as she tried to compose herself.

Zoe had told her that the man was handsome, and she was undoubtedly right about that. His thick brown locks were trimmed neatly and his strong jaw sported a light stubble. His T-shirt was snug, hinting at the defined muscles hidden beneath the material.

But it wasn't Mike's outward appearance that attracted her to him. It was more the kindness in his eyes and his warm smile that made her want to find out more about this stranger.

"I saw your son playing out in the yard earlier today. How old is he?" she asked conversationally as they sat at the breakfast bar with their drinks.

"Curtis is five, and getting to that mischievous age," he said, smiling.

"I'm an elementary teacher, so I'm used to it."

"Really? Curtis goes to Sparrow Falls just a few blocks away."

"Yes, that's where I start teaching next semester."

Mike burst into laughter, shaking his head before catching his breath and explaining,

"Sorry, it's just that I know Curtis will love meeting you. He will take great pleasure in escorting you around the school on your first day."

"Well, I look forward to it," Sarah replied.

She could see the pride in the father's eyes when he spoke of his son. But when the conversation moved on to his work as a mechanic, she could also hear the passion in Mike's voice.

Usually, when Sarah met her pupils' parents, it was when they were stressed, flustered and complaining about their long hours. Mike Jackson, on the other hand, spoke so positively about life - it was refreshing.

The loud ring of his cell unexpectedly interrupted their conversation. His expression turned to one of concern when he saw the number and answered the call quickly.

Sarah waited in silence while he listened to the voice at the other end for a couple of minutes, finally saying, "Right, I will be right there," before hanging up.

His face was apologetic as he turned to her.

"I'm sorry, but Curtis has been taken ill. It's nothing serious; he's just not feeling well. So, I need to go and pick him up."

"No, it's fine, honestly. The poor thing," Sarah smiled.

She couldn't help being a little disappointed as she followed him to the front door. They had been sitting and talking for over an hour, but the time had passed so easily. He appeared just as reluctant to leave when he looked down at her and suggested,

"Perhaps we could do this again sometime?"

"That would be nice."

Sarah waved as Mike went off to collect his son. However, before she could close the door, she spotted Zoe dashing across the road. It was apparent that she had been to the sports club as she still wore her tennis whites. The outfit complemented her tanned, slender figure. Although, her face seemed a little flushed as she gasped…

"Was that Mike Jackson I just saw leaving your house?" Zoe asked.

"Yes, it was," Sarah said gently sighing, knowing that she would now have a barrage of questions fired at her. Yet she found that she didn't really mind. She'd had a circle of friends back in Michigan, but no one that she was particularly close to. So, it was nice to meet someone new, whom she could confide in.

"He saved me from a box that was about to fall on top of me," Sarah explained, as she waved Zoe inside.

"And wasn't I right about how gorgeous he is?" enquired Zoe, with a big smile.

"Zoe, please. I've already told you, I'm off men at the moment" Sarah implored.

However, despite denying her interest in men, Sarah found herself thinking about Mike when her new friend left a few hours later. She found herself secretly hoping that it wouldn't be long before she could spend some more time getting to know him.

Chapter 3
A Heart-Warming Meeting

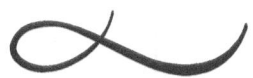

A COUPLE of days later, Sarah was tucking into a tasty turkey wrap. She liked to eat healthily and always tried to visit the gym at least a couple of times a week. Exercise however, was the last thing on her mind today. Instead, she was thinking about her neighbors next door.

Since Mike left the other day to collect Curtis, she had seen and heard nothing of them since. So she was growing concerned about just how sick the boy was and if they needed anything.

"Come on, Sarah, you barely know the guy! He might not appreciate you appearing at his door when his son is unwell," she thought to herself.

The sudden sound of her phone ringing, distracted the young woman's thoughts. As she picked up her cell phone, she smiled when she recognized her mother's number flash on the screen.

"Hi, Mom," she chirped.

"Hello, Sarah. I'm just calling to let you know that your father and I are back home."

"But I didn't think you were due back until Friday?" asked Sarah.

"Oh, I'd had enough of listening to the women constantly competing with one another. Which family has the most money, the most expensive car and the most glamorous vacations? Comparing clothes, and even their jewelry. It was shameful, and I couldn't bear it any longer. So I got your father to order us a charter flight home."

Sarah grinned while rolling her eyes. Her mother had been born into a wealthy family. Her grandfather established a successful company that also sponsored the local university, meaning that she probably had more money than any of the women on the cruise they had returned early from.

However, she was always humble about her family's wealth, preferring to earn her own salary working as a teacher at the university. It was there that she had met her husband, Sarah's father.

After years of helping their students and saving every spare penny, Sarah's parents both retired from their teaching roles early, determined to spend more time together and to travel the world. Leaving their daughter hopeful she would be able to do the same one day.

"Anyway, never mind all that," her mother continued. "As we are back early, your father and I were wondering if you would like to come to brunch on Friday?"

"I would love to," replied Sarah.

"Then you can tell me all about the new house and what your neighbors are like" added her mother.

They spoke for a while longer before arranging a time for her visit. But her mother's mention of the neighbors only reminded Sarah of Mike and Curtis.

"I know what I can do," she declared aloud, rising from her seat.

With that, she dashed through to the kitchen and began busying herself, singing a song that she recalled from her childhood with a soft smile on her face.

Whenever they baked together, Sarah's mother would sing those same words. And that was just one of many happy memories that she had of growing up.

Even though both her parents had hectic careers, they never turned away from spending time with their one and only daughter. So, remembering those years as a little girl was always filled with fondness.

The kitchen was now filled with the aroma of freshly-baked cookies. A loud bleep from the timer indicated that they were ready.

Knowing that the tray would be hot, Sarah pulled on an oven mitt. Opening the door, she felt the intense heat before taking the cookies out and then sliding them onto a wire rack so they could cool.

After filling a plastic container with the warm goodies, she prepared a small flask with strawberry milk. She briefly checked her reflection in the hall mirror, straightening the straps of her floral dress before heading out the door.

However, her original confidence wavered when Sarah realized that there was a second car in Mike's driveway.

"It already looks like they have company. Perhaps I should just come back later," she thought to herself.

Before she could make a hasty retreat, Mike stepped out the front door. He was followed by a tall, thin woman with spectacles that she pushed back up her nose. She wore flat sandals, a loose-fitting skirt, and a top with a love heart logo. Her long brown hair was tied in a tight ponytail that hung to her shoulders.

"Oh, it seems I'm interrupting something," thought Sarah as she watched them exchange a kiss on the cheek. Yet there was nowhere for her to hide as Mike spotted her and called out, "Hi, Sarah."

Feeling somewhat awkward, she approached the pair, forcing a smile as Mike introduced her, "This is Jennifer. Curtis' Mom."

The two women smiled and nodded at each other politely as Mike continued to explain, "Jen, this is Sarah Willis; she's just moved in next door."

" I see that you already have the poor woman baking for you," Jen scolded playfully while motioning to the tub Sarah carried.

"Oh, I just made these for Curtis. That is if he's well enough to have them," Sarah answered hurriedly.

Now both parents burst into laughter, and Jen's almond eyes twinkled as she said, "Well, I'm pretty sure that he will make a sudden and miraculous recovery as soon as he smells them."

Watching them together, Sarah could see how close Mike and Jen were as they shared a final embrace, making her wonder if maybe there were still some romantic feelings between them.

"It's been lovely to meet you, Sarah. Sorry, but I really have to dash. Listen, thank you again for keeping Curtis this weekend, Mike," Jen added as she climbed into her car. "It means that I can do some more work on my case before the big trial next week. I will call later to see how he's feeling."

With one last wave, she pulled out of the driveway and Sarah accepted Mike's invitation to go inside.

"Sorry about Jen," he apologized. "My ex-wife is something of a whirlwind, forever rushing from one place to the next. Her job as a lawyer, I guess."

They had walked through to the kitchen, a much grander space compared to what Sarah had at home. Here, there was every appliance imaginable, with numerous units for storage. All were complemented by marble counter-tops that surrounded the room.

"Like I said, I just brought these for Curtis," said Sarah.

"To be honest, he's just fallen asleep."

Mike must have noticed the disappointment in Sarah's eyes as he was quick to suggest, "But I will be waking him in half an hour. You're welcome to keep me company until then and meet him for yourself."

"I would like that," she admitted.

Opening the door to a drinks cooler, he took out two cans of Coke, chuckling as he popped the ring.

"After a visit from Jen, I usually need one of these as a pick-me-up," he said while filling the first of two glasses. "She certainly makes her presence felt and it helps me relax and finally take a breath once she has gone.

"How did you two meet?" asked Sarah.

Mike took a sip of his drink, while considering the question and then continued. "We met in college, actually. We were both studying law at the time. Jen was always the ambitious one, driven to succeed. We hit it off pretty quickly, but things got complicated when we graduated and started our careers. We were young and had different ideas about where our lives were heading." He paused, reflecting on the past. "But we always had Curtis. He was the best thing to come out of our relationship."

Sarah nodded and took her drink, happy to listen as Mike continued, "I don't mean any of that in a bad way, of course. I have known Jen most of my life, and she has always been the same."

"I'm sorry it didn't work out," said Sarah.

"Don't be" he beamed. "Jen and I are still the best of friends. We just realized that we wanted different things in life. Curtis is the main priority for both of us, and us divorcing amicably while sharing custody was the best solution for him."

"That's wonderful," she commented sincerely. "I have met so many divorced parents over the years and they are usually at each other's throats."

A small voice called from the lounge, "Daddy."

"I bet the smell of those cookies has woken him up," Mike whispered with a wink.

Carrying the goodies, Sarah paused by the door. Mike knelt by his son, who was curled on the couch under a light blanket. Stroking back wisps of the boy's mousy brown hair, he kissed his forehead lightly.

"Hey, I thought you were having a nap, buddy?"

"My nose wouldn't stop wiggling and it woke me," Curtis replied.

His father rested back on his heels, a broad grin on his face as he asked, "And what was making your nose wiggle?"

Sarah remained silent as Curtis gazed up at his dad innocently. His chocolate brown eyes were wide as he exclaimed, "I can smell cookies."

Unable to contain her laughter any longer, Sarah stepped forward to reveal herself. The small boy was eyeing her a little nervously, but Mike was quick to reassure him as he squeezed his hand.

"You're right, this is Sarah. She lives next door now," said Mike.

"Hi, Curtis. I heard you weren't feeling very well, so I baked you some cookies," said Sarah in a friendly voice.

Initially, the little boy's face lit up, until he noticed the flask Sarah held. His expression rapidly changed to one of suspicion.

"What's that? I don't want any yucky medicine," said Curtis as he cringed away in disgust.

"No, this is a special drink. It's a secret recipe that restores your strength and makes you feel better," said Sarah with a smile.

She unscrewed the flask's lid, leaning forward so Curtis could take a tentative sniff.

"It's strawberry milk!" he giggled.

"Because only a few people know how to make it, we must disguise it as something ordinary. But if you drink this, it will take away that icky feeling in your tummy" Sarah explained.

Now that Curtis was content, Sarah joined Mike and his son on the couch. The cookies and milk were soon demolished, although she hardly noticed as the three of them laughed and joked together for the rest of that afternoon.

Chapter 4
A Day to Remember

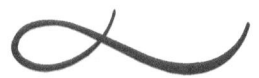

WHEN Sarah woke up on Saturday morning, an orange sun was rising above the distant rooftops. She slipped into her robe and shuffled down to the kitchen, placing a hand over her mouth to hide a yawn as a pot of coffee began to brew.

She had enjoyed a lovely brunch with her parents the day before, listening to their tales about the latest cruise while her Mom scrolled through numerous photos on her cell phone.

When she returned home, she began preparing some lesson plans for her first day at the new school the following Monday.

Waking in the early hours of Sunday with her head on the desk and a painful ache in her neck, she scolded herself, "Come on, Sarah! You need to wake yourself up. You made a promise to Curtis."

It was right, and she was determined not to let the little boy down. A tender look crossed her face as she thought back to the day when she had taken the cookies and milk round.

Curtis had pleaded with her and Mike for them all to go on a picnic together at the weekend as Sarah got up to leave. Her cheeks had turned a pale shade of pink, but she couldn't resist his hopeful stare and eventually agreed to join them.

Mike insisted that he would organize the fried chicken and coleslaw, leaving Sarah to sort out a pasta salad and some tasty desserts. So, after turning on the oven to preheat, she began to collect the ingredients she needed to make some muffins.

While the muffins baked, she leapt into the shower, dressing afterwards in some linen pants and a thin top. The weather was still hot, but they would be exploring the woods, so she knew she needed to keep her legs covered.

A short time later, she knocked on Mike's door, a picnic hamper filled with food and drink hanging on her arm. They welcomed each other warmly as he ushered her across the threshold.

"I've got this to carry everything," he said, sounding rather proud as he pointed at the backpack on the kitchen table.

Sarah had never seen anything like it. Zipped side pockets held everything you could possibly need for a picnic. There was cutlery, crockery, and even tiny salt and pepper pots, along with plastic glasses for drinks.

There were also ample separate sections, all with cooling linings to store their food. Once they were filled, the three of them set off toward the woods.

As they strolled along, Curtis chatted constantly. Due to her teaching, Sarah had instantly noted the boy's hyperactivity the first time they met. So she remained patient while absorbing his every word.

"You really have a knack with him," Mike observed when his son ran off ahead.

"It's my job," she answered casually.

"Perhaps, but he has certainly taken a liking to you," commented Mike.

"And me to him," she said.

She was being honest but also felt shocked to admit it. This was only the second time they had met, yet she felt strangely protective of the five-year-old.

"I'm relieved to know that you will be there at the school watching his back. The teachers do their best, but as you can see, he can be a handful," Mike admitted.

By now, they had reached the first bank of trees in the woods. Paths led off in numerous directions, but Curtis instinctively turned to the right.

Mike and Sarah were close behind, grateful for the leafy arch of branches overhead that shaded them from the day's heat.

"How does Curtis cope in class?" Sarah asked.

"Apparently, he is doing very well. His teacher seems able to calm him easily and refocus him on the lesson. But I can appreciate that he must be hard work for them."

"We do get basic specialist training so we can deal with students who have greater needs or have problems keeping focused. He's so adorable, though; I don't see how anyone could resist him."

Curtis was hunting through a bed of clover, looking for the lucky one with four leaves. Sarah and his father watched from perched tree stumps nearby.

The young woman welcomed the break, pouring drinks of lemonade after trying to cool herself with a weak wave of her hand.

"I'm surprised he can even remember the way through all these different paths," Mike suddenly commented.

She stopped with a glass in mid-air, waiting for him to explain his comment further.

"You see, Jen and I used to come out here most weekends, but Curtis was just a baby back then. So how does he know?"

"It's a mystery," Sarah replied with a spooky tone to her voice.

Awkwardly smiling and rolling his eyes in response to her joke, Mike stood, calling to his son. Feeling guilty for her jocular response, Sarah rose and touched his arm gently. He placed his hand over hers, his brown eyes light as he reassured, "Don't worry. Come on."

They continued picking their way through the lush undergrowth until Curtis squealed with delight.

"Look, Daddy, I found it."

Stepping into a small clearing hidden among the thick trees, Sarah understood why Mike's family had escaped here. It was so peaceful, with only the birds chirping their song in the background.

Lifting his son high into the air, Mike cried out, "Yes, you have my clever boy!"

The sight of them was so rewarding, warming Sarah's heart. She had to admit that the place was beautiful.

Her nostrils were filled with the scent of wildflowers, their beautiful colors contrasting against the lush green grass. Sunbeams filtered through the high leaves, casting light shadows upon the ground.

Curtis ran off to explore while Mike laid out a checkered blanket. He and Sarah sat beside each other, enjoying the quiet for a moment.

"This place must have been very special to you and Jen if he remembers it so clearly," she eventually commented cautiously.

"No, not at all," he corrected her. "When he was younger and while Jen studied to become a lawyer, I would go on long treks. I always took Curtis with me, carrying him on my back in a knapsack.

"We would explore everywhere and could be gone for hours. One day, I just came across this place. The next time we ended up here, Jen was with us, I told her I had never been here until then."

"You lied? Wow!" Sarah was really surprised.

Mike looked at her sheepishly as he begged, "Please don't ever tell Jen that. I made out that we found the place together so that it could be a special spot for her and our son. She has always felt guilty about not spending enough time with Curtis because of the job. I wouldn't do anything to hurt her because I know how much she loves him."

"Of course not, I understand" Sarah replied.

Sharing a secret that he had kept for so many years filled Sarah with appreciation that he felt able to confide in her. Yet she silently cautioned herself, "Slow down, lady, you do this every time. Stop rushing in and making a fool of yourself. Just take a step back for a change!"

When he gently touched her hand and thanked her, she couldn't prevent the fluttering in her stomach. "Thank you."

"You did a very thoughtful thing, so you don't need to worry about me revealing your secret," she replied softly.

Mike's expression as he looked at her echoed his gratitude, without him uttering another word. However, a call from Curtis broke their eye contact, leaving Sarah to watch as Mike began to chase the young boy. She laughed to herself when she heard his childish giggles.

Soon, she became involved in their game of chase when Curtis suddenly ran over to where she sat, trying to hide behind her for protection while his father loomed down on them.

Quickly, she jumped to her feet, taking Curtis' hand and running away with a joyous squeal. Mike was close behind as they tried to escape and not get caught.

After a while, he gained ground and reached out an arm, causing the three of them to tumble to the ground.

Sarah gasped for breath, her stomach now aching from all the laughter. She turned her head, seeing Mike squeezing his son tight before showering Curtis with kisses.

The sight warmed her heart and she began to wonder what it would be like to be a part of this small family. Imagining tucking Curtis into bed every night and taking him to school the next day. The thought of being part of this family made her heart begin pounding in her chest. It was nothing more than a dream.

Chapter 5
A Surprise Invitation

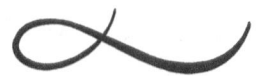

FOR THE next couple of weeks, Sarah spent more and more time with Mike and Curtis. They ate at each other's houses, went on day trips together, and even had movie nights where they would all cuddle together on the couch.

Zoe constantly teased Sarah about it all, leaving the young woman flushed while she tried to deny her true feelings. In reality, she was growing to love and care for the father and son more with each passing day.

Today, however, her stomach was knotted with nerves, and she paced the lounge floor while waiting for her friend.

It was a total shock to her the other night when she left Mike's house. The rom-com had ended and it was getting late. Curtis was already fast asleep in his bed.

However, as they lingered at his front door, Sarah sensed that Mike wanted to say something.

Her mouth fell open with surprise when he suddenly asked, "Sarah, would you consider coming on a date with me Saturday night?" Her bright blue eyes were wide, stunned by the invitation, and she answered with a gasp, "I would love to."

Once she got home that night, though, she immediately called Zoe, suddenly feeling panicked and pleading for her help to get ready for the night.

She was now relieved that her friend had burst into the house, declaring loudly, "Right, let's get this princess ready for the ball!"

"Oh, don't!" Sarah groaned as they both went into the main bedroom. "I'm already a bag of nerves."

"Why? You've been out with Mike plenty of times," Zoe reasoned as she flicked through the hangers in the closet.

"Yes, but Curtis has always been with us. Tonight, it will be just him and me."

"And what's wrong with that exactly?" Zoe asked as she turned to look at her.

Sarah looked down, sighing in exasperation.

"What if we can't find anything to talk about? What if I bore him? I mean, I don't exactly lead an exciting life."

"Don't be silly. Look, the pair of you have loads in common. So stop overthinking things and just be yourself" Zoe said, supportingly.

After a moment's thought, Sarah had to agree. It was foolish to think such a thing. They had never struggled to talk before; why should tonight be any different?

Zoe's positive mood became infectious as Sarah joined her to choose a dress to wear. Finally, opting for a short silver number with matching strappy heels, the outfit accentuating her slim figure and shapely legs.

With her makeup and hair done, she was ready when Mike knocked on her house door a couple of hours later. Now that

Sarah was alone, she needed to take a deep breath before answering it.

He stood there on the step, dressed in a pair of beige slacks and a smart black shirt that was unbuttoned at the collar. His hair was combed neatly, and she caught the scent of his masculine cologne.

"Wow! You look stunning," he gasped.

Sarah was shrouded in the hall light, which caused the gems in her earrings to sparkle. A similar styled pendant hung delicately around her slender neck and a bracelet dangling from her wrist twinkled as she locked the front door.

She blushed while whispering her thanks, feeling the butterflies flutter in her stomach as he offered her his arm and led her to his car.

Following a short drive, they arrived at an Italian restaurant. Sarah gasped in awe when they walked through the grand oak doors. It was like walking into a different world.

Her heels clicked as she walked across the varnished dark wood floor, which ran throughout the building. Already, the aromas of herbs and spices wafted into the foyer area to greet them.

Each wall was adorned with family photographs, showcasing all the people who had been devoted to the place over the years. They hung against backgrounds of eggshell or contrasting red.

The dining room buzzed with activity and the atmosphere was vibrant as they were escorted to their table. Mike pulled out Sarah's chair with a gentlemanly air, leaving her only able to nod politely.

"Everything feels so romantic," she thought. "But come on, girl, you need to keep your cool. Don't get all gushy on me now."

Once they were seated, a sommelier hurried over and promptly offered them a glass of complimentary wine. Sarah eyed Mike over the rim of her glass as she sipped delicately.

"Thank you for inviting me out this evening," she said.

"You have been so wonderful with Curtis over these past weeks. I wanted to repay you for your kindness," Mike replied earnestly.

A candle sat in the middle of the table, its flame appearing to dance when reflected in Mike's eyes. They exchanged a smile, their eyes locked on one another. However, they both quickly averted their gaze when a waiter came to take their order, and Sarah felt the heat rise in her cheeks.

She opted for the venison, with sides of crushed potato and seasonal vegetables, while Mike chose the steak and asked for it to be cooked medium rare. They waited patiently as the sommelier chose the perfect bottle of red wine to complement their meal.

As he popped the cork and poured their drinks with a flourish, Mike asked, "So, how is Curtis doing in school?"

"Really well, all the teachers adore him," Sarah replied.

"That's good to hear. I find myself worrying about how he copes sometimes," Mike admitted.

"Well, there is no need. He is happy and has a lot of friends. And he does seem to be focusing better since you signed him up for the Scouts," Sarah reassured him.

"I hoped it would be good for him. You know, bring him some more structure into his life and to learn things like survival skills in the outdoors," Mike reasoned.

"You can rest assured, it's working wonders already. We have all noticed an improvement in Curtis' behavior," Sarah added.

She leaned across the table and gave his hand a light squeeze. "Mike, you are doing a great job with him."

Seeing the appreciation on his face warmed her heart. She had never imagined that she would develop such strong feelings for Mike and his son. After spending so much time with them recently, she often wondered what life would be like if they were together as a family.

After their food was served, they chatted happily while eating. Their laughter often caused other diners to look in their direction, but neither of them noticed. It was as if the couple were lost in their own private world.

Over an hour later, after Mike had paid the tab, they climbed back into his car. However, instead of heading home, he drove them to a local beauty spot, parking on a cliff top where waves rolled onto the shore below.

It was still early, but the sky was beginning to turn different hues of reds and oranges as the sun sank lower on the horizon. With the car windows lowered, they could hear the sound of the ocean as they both looked out over the expanse of the blue waters.

A balmy breeze tugged at strands of Sarah's long blonde hair. The aroma from the nearby flowers filled her lungs as she inhaled deeply.

"This place really is beautiful."

"It's a magical place. I love just parking here and getting lost in my own thoughts while looking at that stunning view," Mike sighed contentedly.

Sarah murmured in agreement, a feeling of peace passing over her as they sat in silence for a while. So she was slightly startled when he gently touched her hand.

"There is something that I need to admit to you," Mike said, lowering his eyes. She could sense his nerves as he battled to find the right words.

"Bringing you out this evening wasn't just as a thanks for everything you have done for Curtis."

"Really?" Sarah kept her tone casual, but inside, her heart was pounding, feeling both anxious and hopeful as she waited to hear what he had to say. Mike turned in his seat to face her with an earnest expression.

"You see, I also wanted us to spend some time alone. Away from Curtis for a change. I'm sorry if that sounds strange, but I've erm…"

Before he finished, Mike leaned forward and kissed her softly on the lips. In that moment, Sarah felt a bolt of electricity surge through her as his hand cupped her cheek.

"Sorry," Mike apologized when they finally parted.

"Please, don't say that," Sarah responded, stroking his stubbled cheek tenderly, her lips meeting his once more. She was barely able to believe his words as he told her, "After the time that the three of us have spent together, I can't deny my growing feelings for you, Sarah."

"I feel the same way too," she whispered.

Now it was Mike's turn to look shocked, but a broad smile soon began to spread across his face.

They fell into each other's arms passionately, and as their kisses grew more intense, Sarah felt the luckiest woman alive to have found Mike and Curtis.

Chapter 6
A Street Celebration

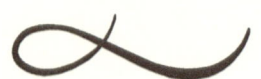

THE NEXT six months were hectic for Sarah. If she wasn't teaching at school, she was either with her parents, her friend Zoe, or Mike and Curtis. She often found herself preparing for Monday morning classes, late the night before. She loved every minute about being so busy.

Her time with Mike and Curtis were always fun -especially as they had decided that it was important for them to show Sarah all the important places in the area. Evenings with Mike were very special. They had returned to his favorite place by the sea several times and had also spent many hours in his back garden with a drink discussing anything and everything. More than once, Sarah had been surprised how easy Mike was to talk to and also how they shared many similar views on so many topics – she could not believe how happy he made her. Even Zoe had noticed a change in her, she exuded a new confidence and contentment with life.

Today, Sarah was helping Zoe and the other women from the street organize a party. One of their neighbors had recently welcomed a new daughter into the family and they were determined to celebrate with everyone to thank them for all the kindness they had shown.

While Sarah helped hang banners and fill balloons, she felt really grateful to have moved there. This was something she had always dreamed of - to be part of a caring community that looked after one another. This was precisely what she had found.

"Sarah – a hand please, quick!" Zoe was heading toward her, struggling with a large crate of drinks. Sarah immediately dashed over to take it, carrying it to the bar area that had been set up at the far end of the street.

"My boys are looking forward to this party today," Zoe commented vaguely. "Did I tell you that they are both bringing their girlfriends?"

"Girlfriends!"

"I know, they are growing up so fast," she said as the women began to lay the long row of tables that had been set up. All the residents had carried out their dining sets, ready for the feast. Numerous barbecues were now lit, warming, ready for the cooking to start. The tempting smell of charcoal filled the air.

Some of the other women were dashing between the houses, collecting the various dishes that had been prepared and placing them on tables that ran along one side of the street so that people could serve themselves.

"Surely it's a good thing that they are bringing the girls to meet you and Tom?" Sarah reasoned.

"It is, but to me, they will always be my babies," Zoe grumbled with a mock pout.

Laughing, Sarah pointed out, "You do realize how silly you sound, don't you?"

After sticking out her tongue playfully, Zoe flounced away to bring more supplies. Sarah shook her head with a smile, although she wondered how she would react in that same situation.

"I mean, I know Curtis isn't my son, but how will it feel for Mike and I when he starts to bring girls home? More importantly, she wondered how would Jennifer react?"

Before she could become absorbed in her thoughts, Curtis ran towards her, calling out, "Sarah, look what me and Daddy have made."

The young boy carried a large tub piled high with brightly iced muffins, grinning as he proudly placed them on a nearby table.

"Wow! They look fantastic," Sarah gushed. "And there's definitely enough there for everyone!"

However, Curtis was already distracted having seen a school friend. He glanced at his father for a nod of confirmation before racing over.

"He has had me up since six this morning baking those," Mike chuckled.

"Oh no," Sarah sympathized with a laugh.

Music started playing from one of the neighbors' homes, adding to the feeling of celebration.

A glorious sun shone brightly overhead as people began to gather for the festivities. The couple for whom the celebration had been organized appeared at their front door.

Katy was blooming as a new mother, holding her daughter closely as if she feared the tiny baby might break. Phil had a hand on his wife's shoulder, beaming with pride as the crowd erupted into cheer, applause and words of congratulations.

However, the smell of cooking soon aroused feelings of hunger in everyone, with a growing line quickly queuing for their food.

Mike and Sarah juggled their plates as they maneuvered back to the table, where Curtis waited patiently. They enjoyed burgers, hot dogs, and charred ears of corn, which they all tucked into with murmurs of delight at the sumptuous flavors.

As she ate, Sarah glanced around her. Everyone was smiling, chatting and seemingly happy to be among friends. The new parents were showing off their baby amid coos of delight from some of the other mothers.

The young woman couldn't have imagined living anywhere more perfect. It was comforting to be living in such a close-knit community, a place where every person in the street was considered with kindness.

Once they had finished eating, Curtis stood before her. She looked at him surprised as he crossed an arm across his torso, bowing slightly as he requested, "Please, could I have this dance?"

"I would be honored," she curtsied.

His hand felt tiny in hers as they moved to a clear space. His stubby fingers barely reached her waist as a slow song began to play. And while they danced, Sarah could hear people's whispers of approval.

"Could I cut in, please?" Zoe wore a flowing floral print dress that swished around her knees as she whisked Curtis away. Yet Sarah was puzzled by her friend's nod until Mike suddenly appeared to tap her on the shoulder.

"Perhaps you would consider dancing with me instead?" he asked.

"Of course," she grinned.

But when Mike took her in his arms, she had to disguise her gasp as a cough. The feel of his hand on the small of her back sent shivers down her spine. She struggled to follow the steps, her eyes intent on his. When the tune finally ended, Sarah was disappointed when he quickly excused himself. Wandering back to their table alone, she took a gulp of soda from her cup. Slumping down into a chair, she sighed heavily.

"Mike has been disappearing a lot lately. I guess he must be getting bored of me already," Sarah muttered to herself, her heart sinking with a familiar type of disappointment. She had been let down by men so many times in the past, so she was waiting for what she thought was the inevitable, when Mike finally returned a short time later.

Her mouth dropped open when he leaped onto the table, spreading his arms wide as he yelled, "Could I have everyone's attention, please?"

Silence fell over the crowd as everyone looked toward him, glancing between themselves curiously as Mike continued, "I know that we are all here today to celebrate Katy and Phil's beautiful new baby, but, there is something that I need to do and I can't wait any longer."

Jumping down from the table, he dropped to one knee, holding out a small blue velvet box while asking, "Sarah Willis, would you please do me the honor of becoming my wife?"

Sarah's blue eyes had been fixed on him, their intense stare hopeful. Suddenly, overwhelmed with joy, she couldn't help but squeal with glee as she happily accepted his proposal.

The cheers and applause that rang out sounded muffled as Mike picked her up by the waist and spun her around.

Sarah was brimming with happiness. Everywhere she looked, she saw smiling faces and heard warm words of joy and congratulations. She was surrounded by so much love. When Sarah suddenly caught sight of Jennifer, she felt a sudden pang of doubt in her heart.

"Don't look so worried," Jennifer whispered to Sarah as she hugged her warmly.

As the party continued around them, Jennifer spoke honestly. "Mike warned me that he was going to propose. I honestly couldn't be happier for you both. Truly."

"Thank you," Sarah answered. Hearing Jennifer's words made her remove any guilt she may have felt in assuming that Mike's ex-wife would be annoyed about her entering Mike's life. But here she was, giving the couple her blessing. With that weight lifted off her, Sarah felt herself relax.

Both women exchanged a friendly peck on the cheek and Sarah could tell that Jennifer was being genuine when she finished by saying, "Seriously, I couldn't think of anyone better than you to become my son's stepmother. Curtis already adores you."

"I adore him too."

It was then that the boy suddenly appeared, his face dirty from grappling with a friend on the lawn. Jennifer hunkered down to his level, and the pair hugged tightly.

"Have you heard Daddy's good news?" he asked matter-of-factually once they pulled apart.

Jennifer smiled softly while answering, "Yes darling, I have. How do you feel about it?"

Sarah held her breath, her thoughts became frantic while she waited for him to reply.

"What if he doesn't want Mike to remarry? What will happen then because we obviously have to take Curtis' feelings into account?" Thoughts raced around her head.

"Oh, it's fine by me. I mean, some of my friends have more than one Mommy or Daddy, and they love it. I will too, especially if I always get extra candy and toys like they do," he finally remarked casually.

Sarah stifled a laugh, Curtis' parents doing the same, as the three of them exchanged a look of disbelief at his cheekiness. The women's expressions soon changed to ones of pleasant alarm when Mike joked, "And just think how clean the house will be with a woman around the place."

Jennifer and Sarah's eyes met and it was as though they knew what the other was thinking. Each grabbed a jug of water from a nearby table and chased Mike as he tried to escape with his son on his shoulders.

The four of them soon collapsed in a heap on a blanket of grass. Once more, Sarah felt fortunate to have found this new life.

Epilogue
Growing Together

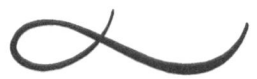

TWO YEARS later, Sarah stood at the kitchen window, watching Curtis play in the backyard. A loving smile spread across her face as she observed him climbing into the tree house he and his father had built together.

Though only seven years old, Curtis displayed remarkable maturity for his age. Despite Sarah's initial reservations about his safety, he had pleaded for his own private space. After numerous discussions and assurances from Mike about the structure's safety, Sarah had relented.

"I suppose I can't blame him," Sarah reasoned to herself. "It won't be this nice and quiet around here for long."

She gently stroked her bulging stomach, aware that her due date was growing ever closer.

Although Sarah considered Curtis to be her son, this would be her first child of her own. The prospect was both daunting and exciting at the same time. However, nerves consumed her when she thought about the night ahead.

Zoe had organized a baby shower for her best friend, but she looked confused when Sarah insisted that the men also needed to be there. Sarah confided that she and Mike would be doing a surprise gender reveal and wanted everyone they loved to hear the news together.

Yet, when she walked through Zoe's garden gate later that evening with her family, all of Sarah's worries disappeared.

Strings of lights adorned the bushes around the seating area's edge, casting a warm glow. A large banner with the word "congratulations" was pinned above the patio doors, welcoming guests inside.

As the doors were opened wide, the dining and kitchen space revealed every surface covered with various platters of food. Friends and family filled the room and Sarah waved back at her parents when she spotted them in the crowd.

Mike guided Sarah through their guests, expressing gratitude for their thoughtful gifts as they made their rounds. Music played softly in the background and some couples began to dance. Sarah was preoccupied with greeting her parents with a warm embrace when they finally found each other in the bustling room.

"You look wonderful! You are literally glowing," Sarah's mother exclaimed with admiration.

"Thanks, Mom," Sarah smiled gratefully. "But I think my flushed cheeks might have more to do with the day's heat."

Her mother tapped her arm affectionately. "Stop it, silly."

Zoe's voice suddenly rang out, capturing everyone's attention. All eyes turned to her as she made an announcement.

"Well, as you all know, Sarah and Mike are going to be having their baby soon. Yet that isn't the only reason why we are all here today. It appears that the pair have something else that they would like to share with us."

Holding hands, the couple moved to stand where they could be seen. Sarah took a deep breath before she began speaking.

"When I moved here from Michigan, my parents had already told me what a wonderful place Weston is. I never imagined that living on this street would help me find the most amazing family in Mike and Curtis. I certainly didn't think I would make such fantastic friendships."

Her heartfelt words elicited murmurs of agreement and nods of understanding from the guests. Sarah paused for a moment, allowing her sentiments to sink in before continuing.

"So, Mike, Curtis, and I have decided that we want all the people we care about here while we do a gender reveal."

Excitement began to buzz through their guests and glasses of Champagne were passed around.

Sarah opted for a non-alcoholic version as Curtis came to stand by them, anticipation written all over his face.

Zoe appeared from inside the house, holding an over-sized helium balloon. Sarah's stomach flipped nervously as she watched it being released. The small family huddled together while the balloon rose higher.

Everyone looked skywards expectantly until a sudden popping sound could be heard. The burst balloon released a shower of pink confetti, and their neighbors erupted into cheers.

Curtis glanced up at Sarah and his father with wide eyes. He had a massive grin on his face as he told them, "I can't wait to be a big brother to my new sister."

Without another word, he ran over to his friends and Sarah smiled as Mike carefully swept her into his arms, placing a loving kiss on her lips. She melted against him, oblivious to everyone else.

"Thank you for making me the happiest man alive," he whispered.

"I couldn't imagine my life without you and Curtis. And now we will have a daughter to complete our little family."

As their lips lingered in another kiss, Sarah sighed contentedly. Moving to Florida had brought her the life she had always longed for. She couldn't think of anyone better to spend it with than Mike and their children.

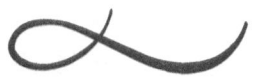

Other Books from Seniorality

To find your next book Seniorality book visit:

www.amazon.com/author/seniorality

Where you will find:

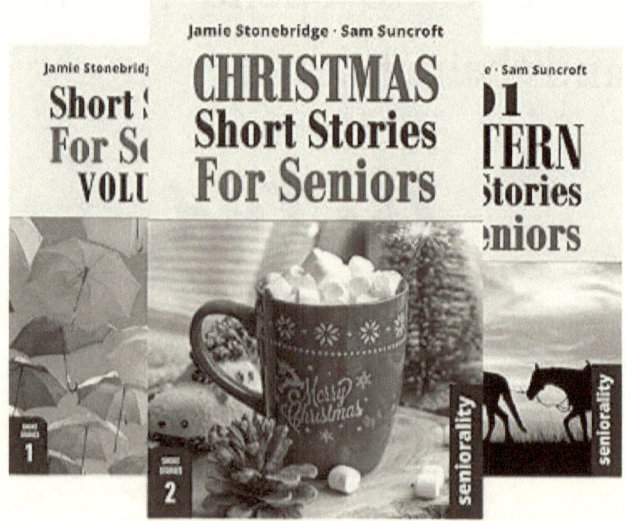

Short Stories

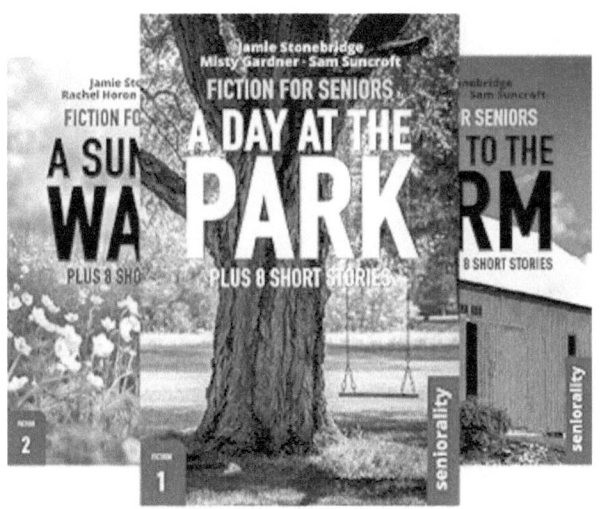

Fiction for Seniors

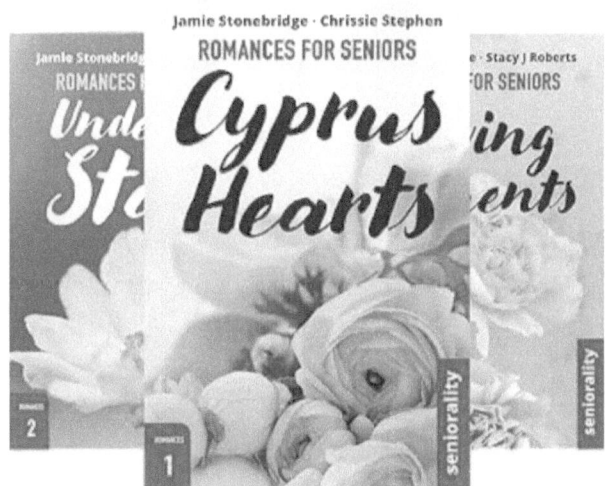

Romances for Seniors

Find these and many more books
by searching on Amazon for 'seniorality'
or visit: **www.amazon.com/author/seniorality**

Thank You

If you enjoyed this book or found it useful, we'd be very grateful if you'd post a short review on Amazon.

Your support really does make a difference and helps other people discover this book.

We personally read all reviews to hear how the books are being used, to collect feedback, and get ideas for future stories.

Thank you and have a wonderful day!

www.ingramcontent.com/pod-product-compliance
Lightning Source LLC
Chambersburg PA
CBHW020437220526
45464CB00002B/750